MILK THISTLE:

THE LIVER HERB

Christopher Hobbs

SECOND EDITION

THIRD PRINTING

Beth Baugh, editor
Virginia Rose Ducale, illustrator

Botanica Press
Box 742
Capitola, CA 95010

Other books available from Botanica Press by
Christopher Hobbs
in the "Herbs and Health Series":

ECHINACEA   The Immune Herb

GINKGO   Elixir of Youth

USNEA   The Herbal Antibiotic

VITEX   The Women's Herb

NATURAL LIVER THERAPY

MEDICINAL MUSHROOMS

FOUNDATIONS OF HEALTH

INTRODUCTION

Medicinal herbs are still used by the majority of the population in the world today for prevention of disease and restoration of wellness. Nine hundred million Chinese people still rely on herbs for a major part of their health care.[1] In the United States herbs have been largely supplanted by chemical drugs, but their use is becoming increasingly widespread due to the popularity of the health food movement.

This booklet will describe one medicinal herb, *Silybum marianum*, that has attracted much interest in recent years, especially in Europe, where commercial preparations are being manufactured for severe liver diseases like hepatitis and cirrhosis, as well as for liver restoration. Our modern environment is full of stressful chemicals, such as food additives and pesticides. These chemicals need to be processed by the liver so that they can be eliminated by the body. Further, the liver is an important organ in the digestion of fat, which is usually over-abundant in the modern diet.

It is hoped that this booklet will increase awareness and use of this herb, which grows commonly as a 'weed' throughout the country.

HISTORY

Through the ages, various thistles have been thought of as part of the ancient curse of civilization and are mentioned as such in the Bible. After Adam and Eve ate the apple, God said: "*Thorns also and thistles shall it bring forth to thee.*"[2] They are a sign of rich land gone wrong. Bristly and prickly, they spread rapidly and cover vast fields. However, thistles can be considered a blessing as well as a curse, for since ancient times, many thistles were widely used for their curative effect on the liver and recently, chemical compounds from the seed of one thistle—*Silybum marianum*, the Milk Thistle—have proven its ability to protect and rebuild the liver.

The ancients revered Milk Thistle. The Greek herbalist, Dioscorides, wrote that a tea of the seeds could be drunk for snake bites.[3] Gerard, the famous English herbalist, wrote: "*My opinion is that this is the best remedy that grows, against all melancholy diseases.*"[4] (Melancholy comes from *melanos*—black and *chole*—bile; an old reference to any liver or bile related disease.) Culpepper thought Milk Thistle good for removing obstructions of the liver and spleen. He recommended the infusion of the fresh root and seeds against jaundice.[5]

The Eclectics, a school of medical herbalists of the late 19th and early 20th century, used it widely for varicose veins and congestion in the pelvis—especially in menstrual difficulty and for congestion in the liver, spleen, and kidneys. They recommended five-drop doses of the tincture three times a day, until relief is obtained.[6] The remedy acts slowly, so it must be taken persistently.
Silybum was also a popular garden plant, valued for its edibility as well as its medicinal attributes.

PHARMACOLOGY
Milk Thistle's long-standing reputation led to production of an herbal preparation for liver-related diseases by Dr. Madaus and Co., in Germany. This, in turn, led to investigation of its efficacy and action by Dr. Magliulo (1973). He demonstrated stimulated regeneration in the livers of rats where this organ was partially removed, when he gave them an extract of Silybum, called silymarin.[7] Silymarin is the collective name by which the primary group of active chemical isomers of Silybum is known. The isomers are silybin, silydianin and silychristin, with silybum, being the most used in clinical applications. The mechanism of this silymarin action was not made clear until 1980, when Dr.

Sonnenbichler, from Munich, showed in *in vivo* tests that silymarin leads to increased protein synthesis in liver cells, due to an increased activity of ribosomal RNA via the nucleolar polymerase A.[8]

Ribosomes are the cellular organelles where proteins are synthesized. There are three enzyme systems in most animal cells to facilitate this process:

- **polymerase A** (transcribing ribosomal genes from DNA, to produce more ribosomes).
- **polymerase B** (for messenger RNA that transfers the genetic information from DNA to the ribosomes where proteins are synthesized).
- **polymerase C** (for transfer RNA which helps connect the amino acids together in the proper sequence to form proteins and enzymes in the cell).

These enzymes and other proteins are integral to the life processes of the cell and ultimately the whole body.

Part of the silybin molecule has a steroid structure.[9] Steroids enter the cell and stimulate the induction of new DNA and ribosomal RNA synthesis. This may be the mechanism by which silybin (a unique kind of flavonoid, called a flavanolignin) works. Flavonoids are very common bio-active compounds. Many of them are plant pigments (rutin from buckwheat is an example). Flavonoids have the basic structure:

The flavanolignans are produced in the plant by a coupling of a flavonoid and coniferyl alcohol. Coniferyl alcohol is a common phenolic compound, widely used by plants as precursors to more complex molecules: the structural material lignin contains many of these units. The structure of silybin is consequently more complex:

Dr. Vogel, a leading researcher of Silybum, has concluded that silybin is a representative of a new class of bio-active compounds. Flavonoids are well known to have blood vessel toning effects, reducing fragility and permeability in them. They also have shown anti-inflammatory effects, but silymarin shows none of these properties. Instead, its action is almost entirely on the liver and kidneys. The evidence for this is that enteral (intestinal) absorption of silymarin is around 50% in humans, renal elimination (via the urine) is slight (5-7%), and the concentration of silymarin in the peripheral blood is slight. Silymarin is subjected to a pronounced enterohepatic circulation (an intestinal to liver loop). It moves from the blood plasma to the bile and is concentrated in the liver cells. This cycle is difficult to break, a reason why some toxic substances (such as a-amanatine, the Amanita mushroom toxin) are so destructive, and why silymarin is so effective.[10]

A-amanatine inhibits the glomerular filtration rate in the kidneys, which results in increased blood concentration of urea and other substances (waste products that can be toxic). Silymarin counteracts this, and the plasma concentration of urea drops.[11] Fortunately, silybin is absorbed slowly when orally administered to various animal species, including humans; and even in large doses, no toxic effects have been noted.[12]

The early groundwork on Silybum by Magliulo, Sonnenbichler, and others has been followed by hundreds of further studies. Representative of this research is Dr. Vogel's work with the most virulent liver toxin known, the above-mentioned a-amanatine from the deadly Amanita mushroom.[13]

Some Amanitas, like *A. phalloides*, (The Death Cup), a common U.S. species, contain two toxins. The first, phalloidine, is a virulent liver poison which destroys the outer cell membrane of the hepatocytes (liver cells), which can lead to death within a few hours. The second, alpha-amanatine, penetrates into the cell nucleus and inhibits the polymerase-b activity, thereby preventing the synthesis of the messenger-RNA, blocking ribosomal protein synthesis and leading to death after 3-5 days.

Silymarin is capable of both preventing phalloidine from reaching its receptors in the membrane (by occupying its binding sites) and transforming the outer hepatocyte membrane in such a way that alpha-amanatine is no longer capable of permeating the membrane. This breaks the enterohepatic circulation of alpha-amanatine, protecting the as yet undamaged liver cells from renewed poisoning. Vogel and co-workers showed that regeneration of a-amanatine-damaged rat livers is accelerated by a factor of four with silymarin, in comparison to untreated controls.[14]

In the 1970s, Vogel conducted a remarkable study. He brought in sixty patients suffering from severe Amanita poisoning from around Europe and treated them with water extracts of 20 mg/kg of silybin a day. Because of humanitarian considerations, no controls were used. Dr. Vogel states that the "results ranged from amazing to spectacular," (all of the patients treated with silybin lived). Even with modern supportive measures (using activated charcoal to absorb toxic-laden bile), the death rate is usually 30-40%.

One remarkable fact was that these patients were mostly treated from 24-36 hours after poisoning, so liver and kidney damage had already occurred.[15] A preparation for injection based on silymarin is now undergoing clinical research by Dr. Madaus Company for cases of Amanita poisoning in humans.

Amanita phalloides is a common mushroom of the West Coast of the U.S. and is increasing rapidly in numbers.[16] It was nearly unknown five years ago, having been introduced from Europe and the Eastern United States, where it is well known.

In the fall of 1983 in the San Francisco Bay area, twenty Laotian refugees were stricken with Amanita poisoning. Several families ate a soup containing the mushrooms, which resembled ones that were considered safe in their homeland; fortunately, they all survived. Since 1981, 36 cases of *Amanita phalloides* poisoning have been reported in the Bay Area alone; five of the victims died.[17] Unfortunately, silymarin therapy has been unknown in this country, but the Poison Control Center in Washington, D.C. has been experimenting with it.

Tests with silymarin have raised other therapeutic possibilities. Recent double-blind studies with cirrhotic patients proved that the survival period was prolonged and the survival rate was significantly increased by silymarin.[18] Other studies have shown liver protection from various other drug and heavy-metal poisoning.[19] See Appendix A for a complete review of scientific findings. The reference list under "General References" is comprehensive.

BOTANY and APPEARANCE

Silybum marianum is a member of the Compositae, the Composite or Daisy family. It is closely related to other thistles, including *Cirsium vulgare* (common thistle), *Centaurea spp.* (Star Thistle), and *Cynara scolymus* (Artichoke). All of the thistles

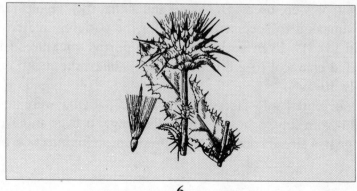

are edible and are known for benefiting the liver,[20] though other than Silybum, none of them are known to contain silymarin.

Silybum is a stout thistle, growing from four to ten feet tall, depending on growing conditions. It has large prickly leaves marked with many undulating white zones. The flowering heads at the end of the stalks are large, bright purple, and beset with an abundance of stout spines.

ORIGIN and DISTRIBUTION

Milk Thistle originates from Western and Central Europe and has made itself quite at home in this country. It was once widely cultivated for its food value and has consequently escaped, now growing wild in many southern areas, including southern Europe, Africa, India, China, and South America. In California, it has been introduced and now grows widely as a weed, especially abundant from the San Francisco Bay Area south to Southern California, thanks to its great distribution system—thousands of parachuted seeds.

It prefers sunny locations, well-drained soil and takes readily to cultivation, though because of its abundance in the wild, it hardly seems worth the trouble for personal use. Milk Thistle has been cultivated in Texas for a large European company and as the demand increases in the U.S., cultivation will become a necessity. It has the advantage, commercially speaking, in being very easy to start, having few predators, and providing a mature crop in less than a year.

Silybum's present growth range is from Vancouver Island to Mexico and east to the Atlantic—though it is less abundant there.[21] It also grows in South America and Australia. In fact, much of the commercial seed production for the European market comes from Argentina.

The plants flower from March in Southern California to July or August in the Pacific Northwest. According to a two-year German study by Voemel in Germany, the southern plants produce the seeds highest in silymarin. The seeds of wild plants from Turkey and Germany were analyzed—the Turkish seeds contained 'markedly higher' silymarin content than the German plants. When wild German plants were grown in Turkey, the silymarin content was higher than normal but not as high as the wild Turkey strains in their native environment.[22] Turkey is about the same latitude as the San Francisco Bay area, Germany about the same as Seattle.

Conditions such as rainfall, average temperature, and the genetic heritage of the plants also affect the production of silymarin by the plant.

COLLECTION

Collecting Silybum is an experience! Find a good population of milk thistle, and bring cardboard boxes, five-gallon buckets, clippers, and most important, thick gloves. Cut the heads with less than 1 inch of stem and place them in buckets, transferring them to the boxes as needed. Look for heads that have finished flowering and are now showing a profusion of white pappus parachutes, for these contain the ripest seeds.

Seed samples from wild California Silybum plants in different developmental stages were sent to Dr. Liersch, Dr.Vogel's colleague from Dr. Madaus Company. His analysis showed the more mature heads contained seeds that had substantially higher silymarin content. According to Liersch, the Silybum seed-vessel, or pericarpium, is the only part of the plant to contain the silymarin (4-6%).[23]

If one waits too long after the heads have opened, some of the seeds will be taken by the wind from the middle of the heads leaving only the seeds around the edge. As many as one-half of the total seeds are lost when the head is past the optimum point. The peripheral seeds seem to be an adaptive feature of the plant. They remain in the heads late into the winter, when they fall and reseed the population. The wind-borne seeds will spread the plants to other areas.

Many species of birds are attracted to the seeds for food. In the

8

summer it is common to see them clinging to the spiny stalks and swaying in the wind as they eat.

RECIPES

The seeds can be ground in a coffee grinder and eaten by the teaspoonful; this is the most delicious and healthful way to add Silybum to the diet. I often pull seeds right from wild heads wherever I find them and chew them up—they are delicious and provide a good taste treat and energy boost.

The kernel itself contains starch, protein and fixed oil. The oil is up to 60% linoleic acid, an essential fatty acid (EFA) needed for prostaglandin synthesis.[24] Recent studies have shown that adding foods rich in linoleic acid to the diet in high enough concentration can reduce chronic inflammation in the body by increasing the synthesis of prostaglandin PGE1.[25] Other benefits of EFA's include helping regulate female hormonal balance, and reducing the possibility of cardiovascular disease, which is still the number one cause of death in this country.

Here are a few other ideas for adding this healthful plant to the diet:

All parts of the plant are edible, especially the young tender leaves and the stalks, which can be eaten raw or cooked. Only the spiny margins of the leaves need to be trimmed away, as they do not grow elsewhere. Silybum has a rich tasty flavor and is quite nutritious. The heads can be eaten cooked like its relative, the artichoke—although with more caution! Finally, the roots may be baked or steamed and taste somewhat like Salsify.

Further ways to use the seeds:

• Soak the seeds overnight in water and puree in an electric blender. Strain off the starch 'milk' and store in quart jars in the refrigerator. This can be drunk by itself or used as a substitute for other liquids in baking recipes. It is high in starch and oil.

9

- Take the drained, ground seeds, roast them in the oven and add salt or herbs to make Silybum gamasio—a seasoning salt.

- Brew the ground seeds with roasted dandelion or chicory to make a delicious hot drink to benefit the liver.

MEDICINAL PREPARATIONS

To maximize the concentration and accessibility of silymarin for medicinal use, make a tincture with the dry, powdered seed. Silymarin is soluble in ethyl alcohol and nearly insoluble in water, so a high percentage of ethyl alcohol to water should be used for the menstruum: 95% if available.[26] Ninety-five percent alcohol is sold in some states under the name "Clear Spring." The tincture should be bright yellow, which indicates the presence of a resinous fraction containing silymarin. The name flavonoid comes from flavus = yellow.

SPECIFIC USES

Specific indications for the tincture are for any liver-based problem: cirrhosis, jaundice, hepatitis, weakened liver from drug or alcohol abuse, or liver poisoning from other foreign chemicals. Congested spleen or lymph can also be benefited, according to the Eclectics. Use it to strengthen the liver, in conjunction with other liver herbs, such as *Cynara scolymus* (artichoke leaves), *Taraxacum officinale* (Dandelion root and leaves), *Artemesia vulgaris* (Mugwort), *A. californica* (Coast Sage), and *A. capillaris* (the Chinese herb Capillaris). *Bupleurum* or *Scutelaria* (Scute), other Chinese herbs, are also valuable.

After several years of using Milk Thistle extract, I have been able to improve my digestion and liver function, which was less than optimum after having hepatitis twice, 20 years ago. I take extra, up to 1 dropperfull of the tincture or 1 tablet of the powdered concentrate 3x a day, when my digestion is feeling weak, for instance, if I experience mild diarrhea or constipation due to overeating, wrong food combinations, eating while tired, etc. This remedy has greatly benefited me and usually brings quick relief, if I combine it with a regime of light eating (mostly fruits and vegetables) for 5 days or a week. Light, circular, clockwise massage of the bowel and liver area is also helpful.

I have also heard some good stories concerning the benefits of Milk Thistle from health professionals around the country. In one case, a woman of 40 was experiencing pain in the liver area, as well as other symptoms of liver imbalance, such as poor appetite and headaches. She went to a medical doctor, who after a series of tests, diagnosed Chronic Active Hepatitis. He mentioned that she should see her banker, a blunt reference to the fact that this was a serious disease. It is worthwhile to note that liver disease is the fourth most common cause of death in this country.

Soon after this diagnosis, the woman heard about Milk Thistle and began taking it daily, 3 or 4 tablets (of the concentrated extract) as well as making some important dietary changes (see dietary recommendations below). Several weeks later she went back for more liver tests and the doctor was astonished to find that the enzyme levels (enzyme tests are one indication of the state of functional balance of the liver) had dropped to nearly normal levels! His only comment was that "there must have been a mistake in the first tests." Two months later I met this woman and she told me that she had been feeling better than for some time. This story is not an isolated incidence, I am happy to say.

One medical doctor I have been in contact with has used Milk Thistle extract in his daily practice for 3 years. He has had good success (up to 50% cure rate) with psoriasis, a disfiguring and uncomfortable skin ailment. He feels that this disease is liver and bowel-related.

Although these experiences are anecdotal, they are about people who have been treated by trained health professionals using modern diagnostic tests. In Europe, Milk Thistle is commonly prescribed by medical doctors for many liver-related imbalances and is a favored medication. It is interesting that from 40-50% of all medical doctors in Germany use phytotherapy in their daily practice.

It seems certain that Milk Thistle and other well-documented herbal remedies, such as Hawthorn and Valerian, will soon take an important place in this country's medicine chest.

DIETARY RECOMMENDATIONS
FOR LIVER AILMENTS

When the liver is under any kind of stress, and especially during specific liver disease, such as cirrhosis or hepatitis, it is important to watch the diet closely. Too much oil and fat, especially when processed or cooked, is hard on the liver. The best oil is olive oil—avoid margarine and animal fat.

Red meat is also hard on the liver, as are drugs of any sort, alcohol, and cigarette smoking. Avoid processed foods generally, and focus instead on whole, fresh vegetables (lightly steamed), whole grains, and slightly sprouted, cooked legumes (such as aduki beans). At least one serving of vital green leafy vegetables a day, such as collards, swiss chard, or beet greens, is highly desirable.

It is fortunate that Milk Thistle has moved to this country and is becoming so abundant and widespread. With drug and alcohol abuse on the rise, and with the number of synthetic chemicals in our environment increasing, our livers are under more stress. As the numbers of Milk Thistles increase, we may be counting our blessings, instead of cursing them.

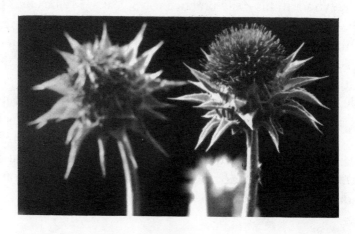

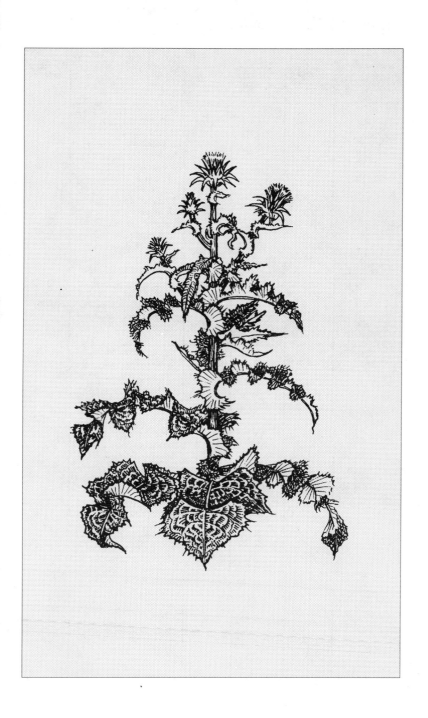

Appendix A: Human Studies

Condition	Duration	Number of Patients	Dosage	Results	References
Chronic alcoholic Liver diseases	6 months	--	--	this double-blind study with histologically proven chronic alcoholic liver disease showed that silymarin was more effective than placebo in enhancing certain immune functions, which may be an important contribution to the liver-protective activity of milk thistle extract; original low T cell and CD8+ counts were raised	Deak (1990)
Toxic liver damage	8 weeks	2,169	--	relief of such symptoms as tiredness, abdominal pressure, poor appetite, nausea, itching	Frerick (1990)
Chronic alcoholic liver disease	6 months	--	420 mg/day	this double-blind trial demonstrated that silymarin (Legalon[tm]) boosted the superoxide dismutase activity of red and white blood cells, as well as other free-radical removing capabilities of various enzyme systems in the body; these positive protective changes were not significant in the placebo group; the researchers theorized that the antioxidant and antiperoxidative activity of silymarin, the main active ingredient in milk thistle extract, may play a major role in its overall liver-protective effects	Müzes (1990)
Hepatits B infection & renal transplantation	--	90	--	improvement of hepatic dysfunction	Chan (1989)

Condition	Duration	Number of Patients	Dosage	Results	References
Chronic alcoholic liver disease	6 months	36	--	patients who were administered silymarin in this double-blind trial showed significant improvements in several liver function tests, as well as histological alterations, over patients in the placebo group not receiving silymarin; the researchers conclude that silymarin was able to "improve liver functions in alcoholic patients"	Feher (1989)
Cirrhosis of liver	2 years	170; 91 alcoholic; 79 non-alcoholic	--	this double-blind study showed silymarin contributed to longer mortality rate, by protecting the liver cells from toxic substances and possibly lessening hepatocellular necrosis.	Ferenci, et al (1989)
Cirrhosis of the liver	41 months	87	140 mg, 3x daily	the mortality rate of patients with cirrhosis (especially alcoholic cirrhosis) was lower where silymarin was administered, and no side-effects were observed	Ferenci (1989)
Type II hyperlipidaemia	7 months (2 month placebo period after the first 3 months)	14	420 mg/day	decrease in total cholesterol, HDL-cholesterol levels, and apolipoprotein levels, with a suggestion of decreased total structural protein amount of HDL, and relative increase in proportion of cholesterol in HDL fraction.	Somogyi (1989)

Appendix A: Human Studies

Condition	Duration	Number of Patients	Dosage	Results	References
Low platelet counts and abnormal liver function tests	30 days	30		this study, with 30 workers who had been exposed to toluene and/or xylene vapours for 5-20 years, showed a significant improvement in liver function tests as well as platelet counts after taking silymarin for 30 days	Szilard (1988)
Amanita poisoning				the use of silymarin alone, or with the addition of penicillin, has been shown to potentially reduce the death rate from ingestion of death cap fungus to 10%	Hruby (1987)
Cholecystectomy	--	6	560 mg;140 mg	when given 560 mg silymarin (silibinin 240 mg=8 Legalon[tm] 70 dragees), maximum serum concentration, as well as renal excretion, were low; however, when 140 mg silymarin (silibinin:60 mg) was given to cholecystectomy patients, maximum silibinin concentrations were found in bile which had been collected from T-tube drains; it was determined that even though the dose was almost four times lower than the previous study, concentration levels were 100 times higher than in the serum.	Lorenz (1984)

Condition	Duration	Number of Patients	Dosage	Results	References
Amanita poisoning	81.6 hours	18	33mg/ kg body weight/ day	this study showed that prevention of severe liver damage is possible, particularly when adminstered within 48 hours after ingestion of *Amanita phalloides*	Hruby, (1983)
Cholecystectomy	3-5 days	11	140 mg t.i.d.	this study showed that biliary elimination of silybinin, the main component of silymarin, occurred no later than two days, and was no longer detectable in the bile after 72 hrs; this indicates therapeutic doses of silybinin can always be detected; however, it does not accumulate in the bile.	Lorenz (1982)
Alcohol-induced liver disease	4 weeks	97	420 mg/day	controlled double-blind study showed 47 patients who were given silymarin experienced the following: normalization of serum transaminases and BSP retention, decreased S-SGPT and S-SGOT, decreased serum total and conjugated bilirubin.	Salmi & Sarna (1982)
Chronic exposure to organo-phosphates			420 mg/day	exposed subjects in the study showed normal values of gamma-GT, LAP, and pseudocholinesterase after the administration of silymarin; those in the non-exposed group showed an increase in gamma-GT and LAP only; there was a marked decrease in serum levels after treatment	Boari (1981)

Appendix A: Human Studies

Condition	Duration	Number of Patients	Dosage	Results	References
Toxic liver disorders		31		in this double-blind trial, the tests of patients with toxic liver damage who received silymarin showed normalcy in a much shorter time than in the placebo group	Fintelmann (1980)
Toxic-metabolic liver damage	2.5 years	--	--	this double-blind study, which was carried out for 28 days for each patient individually, showed significant improvement over the placebo in laboratory findings, including average values for LAP and alkaline phosphatase, which were within normal range	Fintelmann & Albert (1980)
Cholecystectomy	--	9	140 mg	the concentration of silybinin was found in concentrations of 10-50 ug/ml, and the elimination of silybinin lasted for an approximate 24 hr. period; it was estimated the amount of silybinin found in the bile was approx. 20-40%.	Flory (1980)
Acute viral hepatitis	3 weeks	57	70 mg/3x daily	double-blind study showed improvement on serum levels of bilirubin, GOT and GPT, and a tendency to regress pathological values when silymarin was used	Magliulo, et al. (1978)
Acute viral hepatitis	--	59	--	shortened treatment time with patients on silymarin, as determined by GPT-levels	Magliulo, et al. (1978)

Condition	Duration	Number of Patients	Dosage	Results	References
Toxic-metabolic liver damage	--	44	--	treatment with silymarin showed improvement of SGOT, SGPT, and BSP (Bromsulphalein)	Brodanova & Filip (1977)
Sub-acute hepatitis	--	27	--	significant improvement in all patients, including 13 patients with previous HBsAG, who no longer demonstrated this after the treatment; bioptically, 5 patients showed improvement in morphological findings	Chlumsky, et al. (1977)
Chronic fatty liver hepatitis, chronic aggressive hepatitis	6 weeks	--	140 mg/3x daily	with the restriction of ethanol intake, there was some improvement, especially in patients with chronic fatty liver hepatitis	Eberhardt (1977)
Cirrhosis, toxic liver tress	1.5 years		210 mg/day	silymarin showed a beneficial effect in the treatment of liver diseases when taken over a long period of time; no intolerances or side-effects were observed	Filip, et al. (1977)
Chronic hepatitis	3 months- 1 year	36		those given silymarin showed some significant histological improvement	Kiesewettr (1977)
Chronic hepatitis	--	36	--	two controlled studies involving 19 patients treated with silymarin and 17 patients treated with placebo showed excellent effects in the silymarin group as determined histologically, and included improved liver biopsy	Kiesewettr, et al. (1977), Milosavl-jevic (1973), Schilder (1970)

Appendix A: Human Studies

Condition	Duration	Number of Patients	Dosage	Results	References
Cirrhosis	--	13	--	all laboratory results showed improvement with significant improvement of SGOT and SGPT	Brodanova & Filip (1976)
Chronic hepatitis, cirrhosis	up to 6 months	72	70 mg 3x/day	patients treated with silymarin showed major reduction of transaminases, GLDH, LAP, and Gamma-GT in those with fatty liver; silymarin was easily tolerated and caused symptomatic treatment as early as 30 days; positive results were observed in liver cell integrity, excretory function, and the mesenchymal reaction	Ravanelli & Haase (1976)
Abnormal liver functions due to psychopharmaceutical drugs	--	37	--	significant improvement in liver functions tests	Saba, et al. (1976), and Filip, et al. (1976; 1977)
Chronic hepatopathies caused by psychopharmaceuticals		19		in this double-blind study, positive changes were observed in major liver function tests compared to the placebo group; the action of silymarin on the cell membrane was shown to be particularly therapeutic	Saba (1976)
Chronic liver disease		34		after administration of silymarin, there was a marked decrease in triglycerides and total lipids, compared to a placebo group; liver biopsies demonstrated improvement of inflammatory and toxic-metabolic lesions	Reutter and Haase (1975)

Condition	Duration	Number of Patients	Dosage	Results	References
Hepatic cirrhosis	--	11	-	this study demonstrated regression of inflammatory changes and regression of toxic-metabolic lesions	Reutter & Haase (1975)
Hepatic cirrhosis	2-5 years	26	--	biochemical parameters improved in the majority of patients	Benda & Zena (1974)
Acute hepatitis	--	40	--	significant improvement as determined by SGOT and SGPT values	Cavalieri (1974)
Silymarin as a liver protectant with anesthesia and pain-relieving drug to xicity associated with gall-bladder removal	--	20 of 52	4 tablets 3 times daily	silymarin seemed to reduce the liver toxicity of pharmaceutical drug administration associated with gall bladder removal, based on a stabilization of liver enzyme levels over controls	Fintelmann (1973)
Acute hepatitis	--	58	--	in this double-blind study, biochemical values returned to normal sooner in the 29 patients who were given silymarin, than those who were given a placebo.	Wilhelm & Haase (1973)
Hepatitis and chronic degenerative liver disease	2 years	43		earlier favorable results from animal experiments are substantiated with these patients treated with silymarin	Zirm (1973)
Abnormal liver function due to psychopharmaco-logical or anticonvulsant agents	--	66	--	the majority of the patients responded favorably to silymarin, with most liver function tests returning to normal; this indicates liver damage due to these agents can be prevented or lessened with the use of silymarin	Kurz-Dimitrowa (1971)

Appendix A: Human Studies

Condition	Duration	Number of Patients	Dosage	Results	References
Alcoholism				in this study serum bilirubin was normalized, general condition improved, and serum transaminase levels were reduced in patients treated with silymarin	Schmidt (1971)
Fatty infiltration of liver		57		a major improvement in liver enzyme activity was found in 20 of 57 patients, e.g. in the normalizing of bromsulphthalein retention and in glutamic-oxalacetic transaminase activity in 20 patients whose only aetiological factor was alcohol; this study points out the need for further work on the therapeutic action of silymarin in toxic liver damage	Fintelmann (1970)
Toxic metabolic liver damage, chronic persisting hepatitis, & cholangitis with pericholangitis	3 months	67	--	after the 3 month period, bioptical examination showed chronic persistent hepatitis to be resolved, histological examination was congruent with decreased clinical chemical findings, and cholangitis hepatopathies showed excellent response	Sarre (1971)
Chronic hepatitis, cirrhosis, toxic metabolic liver damage	1+ year	43	--	significant improvement as indicated by liver cell permeability, metabolic efficiency of the liver, and excretory function.	Hammerl, et al. (1971)

Appendix A: Human Studies

Condition	Duration	Number of Patients	Dosage	Results	References
Chronic hepatitis, cirrhosis, toxic-metabolic liver damage	5-6 wks. up to several years	2000	35 mg./ 3 x daily	rapid signs of improvement in patient's overall general condition, such as relief of bloating, abdominal pressure, etc., and autonomic symptoms (general weakness, nervousness, insomnia, exhaustion, cardiac pain), increased exercise capacity, improved appetite and body weight gain; in 50-90% of the cases, palpation of the liver supported this, and, in most cases, there was a tendency for the enlarged spleen to shrink; no harmful side-effects were noted.	Holz-gartner (1970), Schopen, et al. (1969; 1970), Jablonska & Reznikova (1970), Marecek (1977), Schmidt (1971), Grosss & Haase (1971), Neumaier (1970), Cuesta, et al., Wilhelm (1972), Zirm (1973).
Acute viral hepatitis	29 days & 43 days	77	--	as determined by GPT-levels, this double-blind study demonstrated 35 silymarin patients needed treatment for only 29 days; in contrast, 42 placebo patients needed treatment for 43 days.	Plomteux, et al. (1971)
Hepatic cirrhosis	--	22	--	SGOT, SGPT, and Serum bilirubin, improved in the majority of cases with silymarin, and most of these returned to normal levels	Hammerl, et al. (1971)

23

Appendix A: Human Studies

Condition	Duration	Number of Patients	Dosage	Results	References
Cirrhosis	4 years	--	-	this double-blind study showed significant lengthening of survival time with silymarin; in addition, with patients who had undergone shunt operations for portal hypertension, silymarin supported liver function, which normally can deteriorate after this type of procedure	Schriefers & Dietz (1969)

Animal and in vitro testing

A large number of animal and *in vitro* tests have also been performed with silymarin, demonstrating a protective effect in isolated animal and human cells, and improvement in a variety of liver function tests after exposure to various liver toxicants. The specific results of these tests will not be quoted here because of the uncertainty of application to humans. For those who find these of interest, a number of the relevant citations are quoted in the General Reference list. A special Symposium proceedings have been published in Germany (Braatz & Schneider, 1976) on the pharmacodynamics of silymarin. These reports are all performed with animal and *in vitro* testing. The individual articles are listed at the end of the General References for completeness.

The author encourages the use of human tests with oral application of natural products and whole herbal extracts as the most effective way to support the long clinical use and history of use of many herbal medicines.

Appendix B:
Commission E Monograph of Milk Thistle seeds.

The following is an official monograph from Germany.

Specification of the medicine
> *Cardui mariae fructus*, Milk Thistle (Mary's thistle) fruit

Composition of the medicine
> Thistle fruit, consisting of fruit (freed of the protective envelope) from *Silybum marianum* (L) GAERTNER as well as preparations in effective dosage (strength).
> The drug contains flavonoid derivatives such as silybinin, silydianin, and silychristin.

Areas of Use
> Drug: Dyspeptic complaints
> Preparations: Toxic liver damage: for supporting treatment with chronicially inflamed liver diseases and cirrhosis of the liver.

Contraindications
None known

Side Effects:
Drug: None known
Preparations: Isolated observations of a mild laxative effect

Reactions with other medicines:
None known.

Dosage
As long as not otherwise directed:
medium daily dosage of drug: 12-15 gm. of preparations:
corresponds to 200-400 mg silymarin calculated as silybinin.

Manner of Use
Ground drug for infusion as well as other preparations from
the drug for oral administration.

Effects
Silymarin has an antagonistic effect against numerous types
of liver injury or damage: poisons of the *Amanita phalloides*
(Death Cap), lanthamden (from lanthanum),
tetrachlorocarbon, galactosamine sulphur acetamide as well
as the hepatotoxic virus FU3 (of cold blooded animals).

The therapeutic effectiveness of silymarin is based on 2
'points of attack' or mechanisms: firstly, silymarin alters the
structure of the outer cell membrane of hepatocytes in such
a way that liver poisons can't penetrate to the inside of the
cell; secondly, silymarin stimulates the activity of the (nucleo-
Polymerase A) with the result being an increased ribosomal
protein synthesis. In this way the regenerating capacity of the
liver is excited and the new building of hepatocytes stimulated.

REFERENCES

1. Committee on Scholarly Communication with the People's Republic of China. 1975. *Herbal Pharmacology in the People's Republic of China.* Washington, D.C.: National Academy of Sciences.
2. *The Bible*, Genesis 3:18.
3. Gunther, R.T. 1968 (1655). *The Greek Herbal of Dioscorides.* New York: Hafner Publishing Co.
4. Gerard, J. 1597. *Gerard's Herbal.* London: John Norton.
5. Culpepper, N. 1847. *The Complete Herbal.* London: Thomas Kelly.
6. Ellingwood, F. 1983 (1898). *American Materia Medica,Therapeutics and Pharmacognosy.* Portland, OR: Eclectic Medical Publications.
7. Vogel, G. 1981. "A Peculiarity Among the Flavonoids— Silymarin, A Compound Active on the Liver." In *Proceedings of the International Bioflavonoid Symposium*, Munich, FRG: 1981, p. 472.
8. Sonnenbichler, J., *et al.*; "Influence of Silybin on the Synthesis of Macromolecules in Liver Cells." In *Proceedings of the International Bioflavonoid Symposium*, Munich, FRG: 1981, p. 477.
9. *Ibid.*, p. 478.
10. Vogel, *op. cit.*
11. *Ibid.*, p. 468.
12. *Ibid.*, p. 463.
13. Vogel, G. 1977. "Natural Substances with Effects on the Liver." In *New Natural Products and Plant Drugs with Pharmacological, Biological or Therapeutical Activity.* New York: Springer-Verlag, pp. 251-265.
14. *Ibid.*, pp. 252-253.
15. Vogel, G. 1981, *op. cit.*
16. Aurora, D. 1980. *Mushrooms Demystified.* Berkeley: Ten Speed Press.
17. Personal communication with the Poison Control Center,

San Francisco, California. (Phonecall, August, 1984).
18. Vogel, G. 1981, *op. cit.*
19. Strubelt, O., *et al.* 1980. "The influence of silybin on the hepatotoxic and hypoglycemic effects of praseodymium and other lanthanides." *Arzneim.-Forsch.* 30: 1690-4.
20. Grieve, M. 1981 (1931). *A Modern Herbal.* New York: Dover Publications, New York.
21. Abrams, Leroy and Ferris, Roxana. 1960. *Illustrated Flora of the Pacific States.* Palo Alto, CA: Stanford University Press.
22. Voemel, A., *et al.* 1977. "The lipid and flavonoid contents in the seeds of *Silybum marianum* Gaertn. under extremely varied ecological conditions." *Z. Acker-Pflanzenbau* 144: 90-102.
23. Szilagyi, I., *et al.* 1982. "Isolation and Structure of Silymonin and Silandrin, two New Flavanolignans from *Silybum marianum* (L.) Gaertn., Flore Albo." *Stud. Org. Chem.* (Amsterdam) 11: 345-51.
24. Voemel, A., *op. cit.*
25. Kunkel, Steven L., *et al.* 1978. "Suppression of Chronic Inflammation by Evening Primrose Oil," *Prog. Lipid Res.* 20: 885-8.
26. Merck and Co., Inc. *The Merck Index,* 9th ed. Rahway, N.J.: Merck and Co. (Silybin).

General References

Bende, L., and W. Zenz. 1973. Silymarin bei Leberzirrhose. *Wiener Medizinische Wochenschrift.* 34-36:512-516.

Benda,L. and W. Zenz. 1974. *Therapiewoche* 24:3598.

Bindoli, A., et al. 1977. Inhibitory action of silymarin of lipid peroxide formation in rat liver mitochondria and microsomes. *Biochem. Pharmacology.* 26: 2405-2409.

Boari, C., et al. 1981. Silymarin in the protection against exogenous noxae. *Drugs Exptl. Clin. Res.* 7:115-120.

Brodanova, M. and J. Filip. 1976. *Prakt. Arzt.* 30:354.

Brodanova, M. and J. Filip. 1976; 1977. Aktuelle Hepatol., *Ber. Symp. Prag.*; Hans. Verl.-Kontor, *Lübeck* S.30.

Campos, R., et al. 1989. Silybin dihemisuccinate protects against glutathione depletion and lipid peroxidation induced by acetaminophen on rat liver. *Planta Medica.* 55:417-419.

Cavalieri, S. 1974. *Gazz. Med. ital.*133:628.

Chan, M.K., et al. 1989. Hepatitis B infection and renal transplantation: The absence of anti-delta antibodies and the possible beneficial effect of silymarin during acute episodes of hepatic dysfunction *Nephrol. Dial. Transplant.* 4:297-301.

Chlumsky, J., J. Filip and M. Brodanova. 1976; 1977. Aktuelle Hepatol., *Ber. Symp. Prag.;* Hans. Verl.-Kontor, *Lübeck* , S. 24.

Commision E. 1986. Monograph of Cardui mariae fructus (thistle fruit). *Deutsche Apotheker Zeitung.* 126.

Cuesta, S., et al. 1973. *Rev. espan. enferm. ap. digest.* 41:87.

Deak, G., et al. 1990. Immunomodulatory effects of silymarin treatment in chronic alcoholic liver disease. *Orvosi Hetilap* 24:1291.

Eberhardt, G. 1977. Efficiency of the healing process in chronic liver diseases. Results of a controlled therapy study. *Therapiewoche.* 27:1944-1946, 1951-1952.

Faulstich, H., et al. 1980. Silybin inhibition of amatoxin uptake in the perfused rat liver. *Drug Res..* 30:452-454.

Feher, J., et al. 1989. Hepatoprotective activity of silymarin (Legalon) therapy in patients with chronic alcoholic liver disease. *Orvosi Hetilap.*130:2723.

Ferenci, P., et al. 1989. Randomized controlled trial of silymarin treatment in patients with cirrhosis of the liver. *Journal of Hepatology.* 9:105-113.

Filip, J., et al. 1977. Further possibilities of the administration of Legalon in the treatment of liver disease. *Verlagskontor Lübeck* . 44-47.

Filip, J., M. Brodanova and J. Chlumsky.1976;1977. Aktuelle Hepatol. *Ber. Symp. Prag;* Hans. Verl.-Kontor, *Lübeck.* S. 40.

Fintelmann, V. 1970. The therapy of fatty infiltration of the liver with silymarin. *Therapiewoche.* 20:23.

Fintelmann, V. 1973. Postoperative behavior of serum-cholinesterase. *Wochenschrift für Klinik und Praxis* 68:809-815.

Fintelmann, V. and A. Albert. 1980. The therapeutic activity of Legalon in toxic hepatic disorders demonstrated in a double blind trial. *Therapiewoche.* 30:5589-5594.

Fintelmann, V. and A. Albert. 1980. *Therapiewoche.* 30:5589.

Flory, P.J., et al. 1980. Studies on elimination of silymarin in cholecystectomized patients. *Planta Medica.* 38.

Frerick, H., et al. 1990. Silymarin-a phytopharmaceutical preparation for the treatment of toxic liver damage. *Der Kassenarzt* 33/34:36-41.

Gross, G. and W. Haase. 1971. *Med. Welt.* 22:1350.

Hammerl, H., et al. 1971. *Med. Klin.* 66:1204.

Hammerl, H., et al. 1971. Über die objektivierung der silymarinwirkung bei Lebererkrankungen. *Med.Klin.* 66:1204-1208.

Holzgartner, H. 1979. *Therapiewoche.* 20:1868.

Hruby, K. 1984. Silybinin in the treatment of deathcap fungus poisoning. *Forum.* 6:23-26.

Hruby, K. 1987. Deathcap fungus poisoning. *Intensivmed.* 24:269-274.

Hruby, K., et al. 1983. Pharmacotherapy of Amanita phalloides poisoning with silybin. *Wiener Klinische Wochenschrift.* 7:1-8.

Jablonska, M. and L. Reznikova. 1976;1977. Aktuelle Hepatol., *Ber. Symsp. Prag.;* Hans. Verl.-Kontor, *Lübeck,* S.48.

Kiesewetter, E., et al. 1977. Results of two double-blind studies on the effect of silymarin in chronic hepatitis. *Leber Magen Darm* 7:318-323.

Kurz-Dimitrowa, D. 1971. Hepatoprotective treatment for neuropsychiatric patients receiving long-term therapy with psychotropic drugs. *Zeitschrift für praklinische Geriatrie* 9:275-279.

Kurz-Dimitrowa, D. 1971. *mda.* 1:275.

Lorenz, D., et al. 1982. Investigations on elimination of silymarin in cholecystectomized patients. *Planta Medica.* 45:216-223.

Lorenz, D., et al. 1984. Pharmacokinetic studies with silymarin in human serum and bile. *Meth. and Find. Exptl. Clin. Pharmacol.* 6:655-661.

Machicao, F., and J. Sonnenbichler. 1977. Mechanism of the stimulation of RNA synthesis in rat liver nuclei by silybin. *Hoppe-Seyler's Z. Physiosl. Chemie.* 358:141-147.

Magliulo, E., et al. 1973. Studies on the regenerative capacity of the liver in rats subjected to partial hepatectomy and treated with silymarin. *Drus. Res.* 23: 161-167.

Magliulo, E., et al. 1978. Zur Wirkung von Silymarin bei der Behandlung der akuten Virushepatitis. *Med. Klin.* 73:1060-1065.

Marecek, B. 1976;1977. Aktuelle Hepatol., *Ber. Symp. Prag* ; Hans. Verl.-Kontor, *Lübeck,* S.74.

Meiß, R., et al. 1981. Ultrastructural morphometric investigation on mouse liver after treatment with phalloidin and a-amanitin followed by application of silybin. *Sonderdruckk-Zeitschrift für Gastro-enterologie.* 8:384-389.

Milosavljevic, Z.1973. *Therap. Gegenw.* 112:968.

Mourell, M. and L. Favari. 1988. Silymarin improves metabolism and disposition of aspirin in cirrhotic rats. *Life Sciences.* 43:201-207.

Mourelle, M., et al. 1989. Prevention of CCL4-induced liver cirrhosis by silymarin. *Fundam. Clin. Pharmacol.* 3:183-191.

Müzes, G., et al. 1990. Effects of silymarin (Legalon) treatment on the antioxidant defense system and lipid peroxidation in patients with chronic alcoholic liver disease. A double blind study. *Orvosi Hetilap.* 131:86.

Neumaier, W. 1970. *Arztl. Praxis.* 21:3637.

Nsassuato, G., et al. 1983. Effect of silybin on biliary lipid composition in rats. *Pharmacol. Res. Comm.* 15:337-346.

Plomteux, G., et al. 1973. *IRCS Med. Science.* 8:259.

Plomteux, G., et al. 1977. Hepatoprotector action of silymarin in human acute viral hepatitis. *IRCS Med. Sci.:Libr. Compend.* 5:259.

Ramellini, G., and J. Meldolesi. 1976. Liver protection by silymarin: In vitro effect on dissociated rat hepatocytes. *Drug. Res.* 26:69-73.

Ravanelli, O. and W. Haase. 1976. The effectiveness of silymarin in diseases of the liver. *Der praktische Arzt.* 30:1592-1621.

Reutter, F.W. and W. Haase. 1975. Clinical experience with silymarin in the treatment of chronic liver disease. *Schweiz. Rundschau Med. (Praxis).* 64:1145-1151.

Reutter, F.W. and W. Haase. 1975. *Schweiz. Rdsch. Med. (Praxis).* 64:1145.

Saba, P., et al. 1976. *Gazz. med. ital.* 135:236.

Saba, P., et al. 1976. Therapeutic action of silymarin on chronic hepatopathies caused by psychopharmaceuticals. *Gazz. Med. Ital.* 135:236-251.

Salmi, H.A., S. Sarna. 1982. Effect of silymarin on chemical, functional, and morphological alterations of the liver. *Scand. J. Gastroentererol.* 17:517-521.

Sarre, H. 1971. Erfahrungen mit Silymarin bei der Behandlung chronischer Lebererkrankungen. *Arzneim.-Forsch.* 21:1209-1212.

Schilder, M. 1970. *Therapiewoche.* 20:3446.

Schmidt, K.H., et al. 1988. Changes in the pattern of microsomal fatty acids in rat liver after thermal injury and therapeutic intervention. *Burns.* 14:25-30.

Schmidt, L. 1971. The treatment of alcoholism and alcohol-induced liver damage. *Therapiewoche.* 21:35.

Schopen, R.D. and O.K. Lange. 1970. *Med. Welt.* 21:691.

Schopen, R.D., et al. 1969. *Med. Welt.* 20:888.

Schriefers, K.H. and D. Dietz. 1969. *Therapiewoche.* 19:1545.

Schriewer, H., et al. 1973. Pharmacokinetics of the antihepatotoxic activity of silymarin in the rat liver intoxicated by CCl4 or deoxycholate. *Drug Res.* 23:157-158.

Schriewer, H., et al. 1975. The effect of silybin-dihemisuccinate on regulation disorders in phospholipid metabolism in the acute galactosamine intoxication in the rat. *Drug Res..* 25:1582-1585.

Somogyi, A., et al. 1989. Short term treatment of type-II hyperlipoproteinaemia with silymarin. *Acta Medica Hungarica* 46:289-295.

Sonnenbichler, J., et al. 1986. Stimulatory effect of silybinin on the DNA synthesis in partially hepatectomized rat livers: non-response in hepatoma and other malignant cell lines. *Biochem. Pharmacol.* 35:538-541.

Szilard, S., et al. 1988. Protective effect of Legalon in workers exposed to organic solvents. *Acta Medica Hungarica.* 45:249-256.

Tuchweber, B., et al. 1979. Prevention by silybin of phalloidin-induced acute hepatoxicity. *Toxicol. Appl. Pharmacol.* 51:265-275.

Valenzuela, A. and R. Guerra. 1986. Differential effect of silybin on the Fe2+ -ADP and t-butyl hydroperoxide-induced microsomal lipid peroxidation. *Experientia.* 42: 139-141.

Valenzuela, A., et al. 1989. Selectivity of silymarin on the increase of the glutathione content in different tissues of the rat. *Planta Medica.* 55:420-422.

31

Vogel, G., et al. 1984. Protection by silybinin against Amanita phalloides intoxication in beagles. *Toxicol. Appl. Pharmacol.* 73:355-362.

Wilhelm, H. 1972. *Zschr. Therap.* 10:482.

Wilhelm, H. and W. Haase. 1973. *Therapiewoche.* 23:3276.

Zirm, K.L. 1973. *Wien. Med. Wschr.* 123:302.

Zirm, K.L.. 1973. The treatment of subacute and chronic forms of hepatitis and of chronic degenerative liver diseases with silymarin. *Wschr.* 19:302-305.

Symposium on the Pharmacodynamics of Silymarin (List of Papers)

Braatz, R. and C.C. Schneider. 1976. *Symposium on the Pharmacodynamics of Silymarin.* Berlin: Urban & Schwarzenberg.

Vogel, G.: Pharmacological properties of silymarin, the antihepatotoxic agent from the seeds of the milk thistle, *Silybum marianum* (L.) Gaertn.

Halbach, G.: Chemistry of silymarin and water-soluble derivatives.

Frimmer, M.: Comparative studies on effects of silymarin in phalloidine action in perfused livers, isolated hepatocytes and isolated membrane systems.

Tuchweber, B.: Modification of experimental liver damage by silymarin.

Braatz, R.: Effects of silybin on phalloidine pre-treated mice.

Kirn, A.: Effect of silymarin on the Frog Virus 3 induced hepatitis in mice.

Trost, W.: Effect of silybin on praseodymium nitrate-induced hepatotoxicity in rats.

Rauen, H.M.: The effect of silymarin N-methylglucamine salt on certain disturbances of phospholipid metabolism of rat liver microsomes after intoxication with thioacetamide, and the influence of silybin hemisuccinate on similar alterations after D-galactosamine poisoning.

Antweiler, H.: Effects of silymarin on intoxication with ethionine and ethanol.

Porcellati, G.: The effect of silymarin on liver phospholipid and protein metabolism in the rat *in vitro.*

Mennicke, W.: What is known about the metabolism and pharmacokinetics of silymarin?

Desplaces, A.: The effect of silymarin on the histochemical picture in normal liver cells and in phalloidine-intoxicated liver cells.

Sieck, R.: Effects of silybin on the LDH of the rat liver.

Down, W.H.: The influence of silybin on the hepatic microsomal drug metabolising enzyme system of the rat.

Schriewer, H.: The effect of silybin dihemisuccinate on lipid metabolism.

Porcellati, G.: The effect of silymarin on biochemical parameters in fatty liver by ethanol.

Seeger, R. The effect of silymarin on erythrocytes.